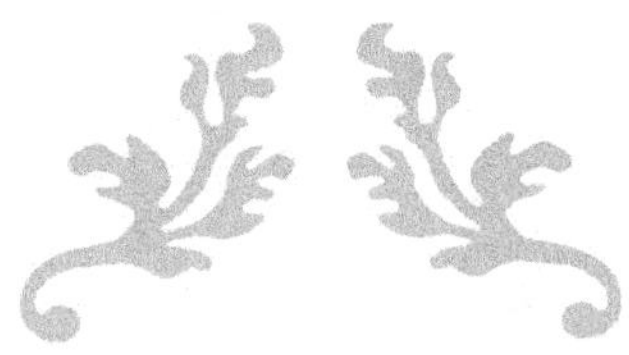

MUSCLE BOUND
MUTHA TRUCKER

How I Build Muscle & Lose Fat While Trucking

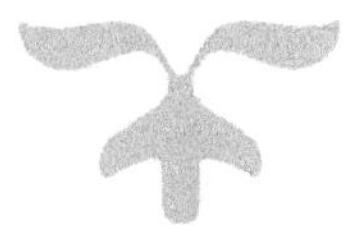

Front cover image by Brian T Westermann

Photos within the book by Brian T Westermann

***** <u>Disclaimer</u> *****

Neither the author or editor, can be responsible for your use of the information contained in these pages of this book. The author or editor assumes no responsibility or liability for any errors or omissions in the content of this book. The information contained in this book is provided on an "as is" basis with no guarantees of completeness, accuracy, usefulness, or timeliness. This book is for entertainment purposes only. Consult your doctor or appropriate health care provider, prior of beginning any exercise program or training. Again, no liability is assumed by the author or editor for the information contained within this book.

What up ….. my name is Brian T Westermann. I have been trucking for about 3 years now with my dog Chloe. It is the simple lifestyle that I enjoy, now that I am 49 years old. Throughout all my years, I have always been fascinated by the strength and muscle development of the top athletes. My first venture into the fitness industry was becoming certified as a personal trainer. It was my first eye opening experience on how people set goals to improve in strength or fat loss, but also how that desire fades quick once they realize the long-term dedication and hard work that is required to reach those goals. Unfortunately, I am not a person that will continually try to motivate another person, so personal training was not for me. Later in life I became a Physical Therapist Assistant, and worked in skilled nursing homes for about 14 years. The COVID situation changed many things within the health industry. After about 2 years of all the changes, I decided to try something new ….. Trucking. Been working at Werner for about 3 years now and I love it !!! The only thing that bothered me was not being able to train with weights anymore. For the first 6 months, I was doing 48 states OTR. Great sight-seeing account, but the scheduling was erratic. Driving drowsy is obviously not the thing to do, so sleep is the #1 priority, and working out was put on the back burner for a while. It has been frustrating for me to not have a set schedule to work out the way I would like and not be drowsy during my drive time. Prior of trucking, I have always had either strength goals, workout progression goals, body composition goals and I also competed in powerlifting.

As C.T. Fletcher would say ….. "I'm an IRON ADDICT". Since I was unable to hit the gym, over time, I created a way to make the truck a portable gym. It took a while to learn how to modify any type of training within the truck. Something always was in the way, the seat back rests for this movement, cabinets for that movement, etc ….. extremely frustrating. I started with bodyweight movements and gradually added my equipment from my storage unit onto the truck. I have modified my equipment and now can train heavy with all movements or body parts, as if I was at a gym. After 2 years of trucking, I did my first strict curl competition. I am close to the world record in my weight class, and will do another strict curl competition once I am able to break that record. When I first started to write this book, it was more of an instructional workout book, but I am just going to state how and why I went about doing things. The world does not need another "know it all" telling people the "RIGHT" way of doing things. On my truck, I have a foldable incline bench that I keep stored on my passenger seat. I have curling bars that are secured to the seat belt harness behind my passenger seat. I have two stacks of weight plates, each on a loading pin in an area underneath the bed that are secured to the structure of the truck. I have multiple TheraBand's with varying resistances. Two sets of adjustable dumbbells (52.5 lbs. & 90 lbs.) from Bowflex. An old-school gadget called the chest expander (oddly enough, it works the back and shoulder muscles). Hand grippers, and various forearm development gadgets. I know it might seem overkill for most, but all this equipment, I already owned.

The exercises and routines I used to stay lean and muscular as a trucker, always changed. Some months, I wanted to focus more on strength or size of a certain body part. Other times, I wanted to be a little bit leaner. Most people who train, usually has a vision of what they want to look like, and/or want to achieve a certain level of strength. There is a universal perception of a male physique called the "Adonis Physique," which I will talk about shortly. The next few pages are pictures of the equipment I utilize, and how I store some of them. The Spud Inc. adjustable front squat harness, loading pin attachments, foldable weight bench, and chest expander can be bought at Amazon.com.

Adjustable front squat harness made by Spud Inc.

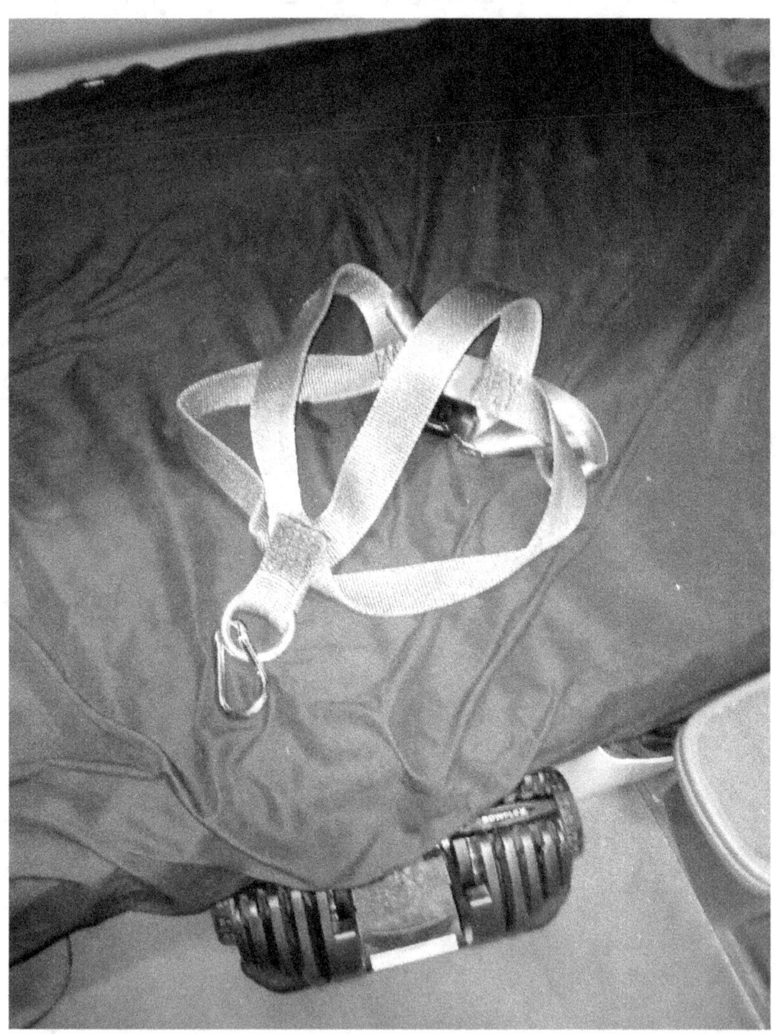

Foldable and adjustable weight bench made by Yoleo

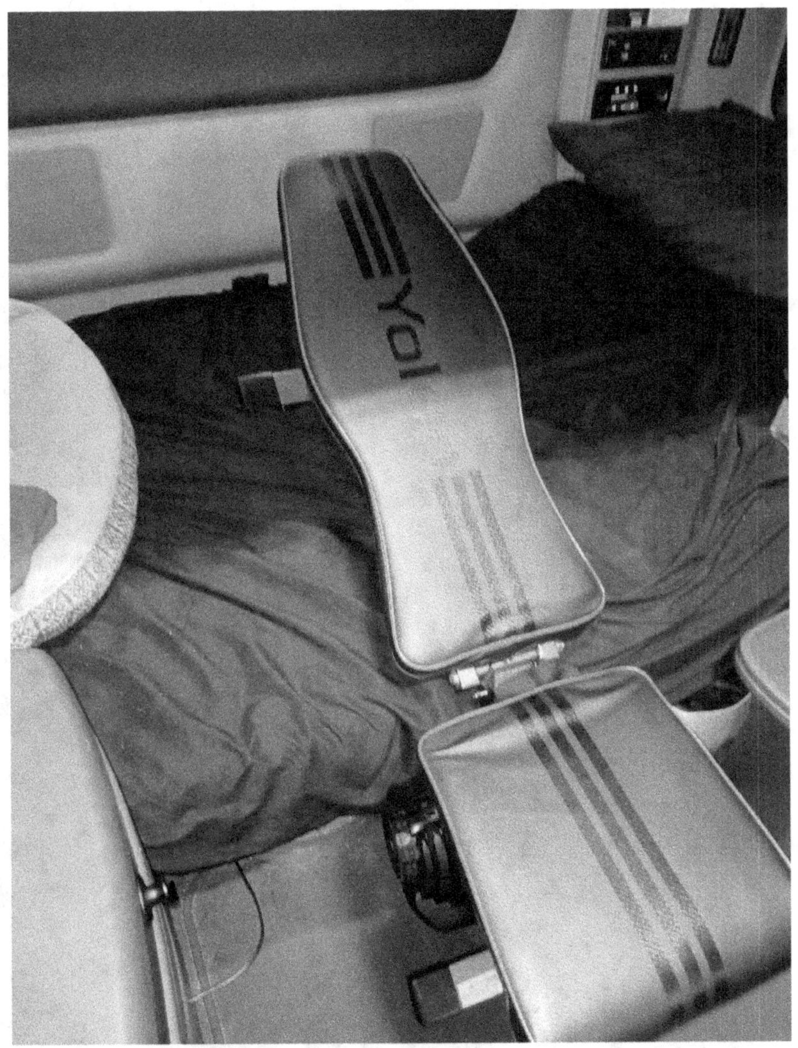

Curling bars are secured to the seatbelt harness behind the passenger seat

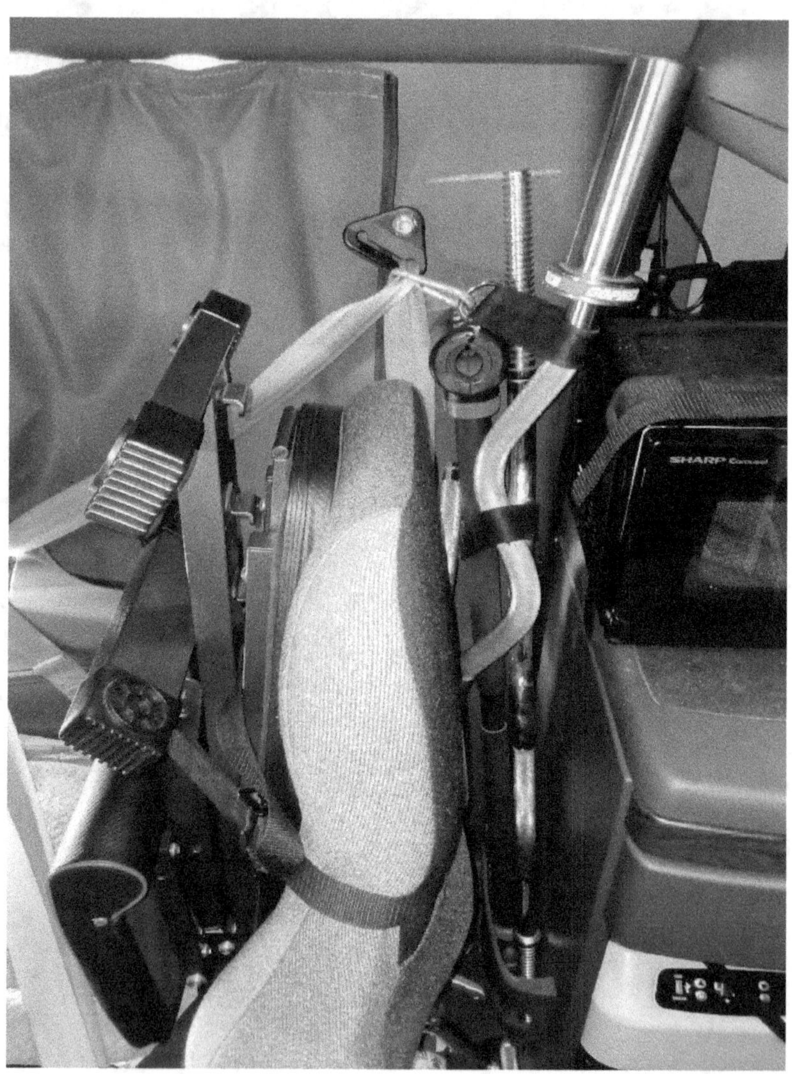

Foldable weight bench secured to passenger seat.

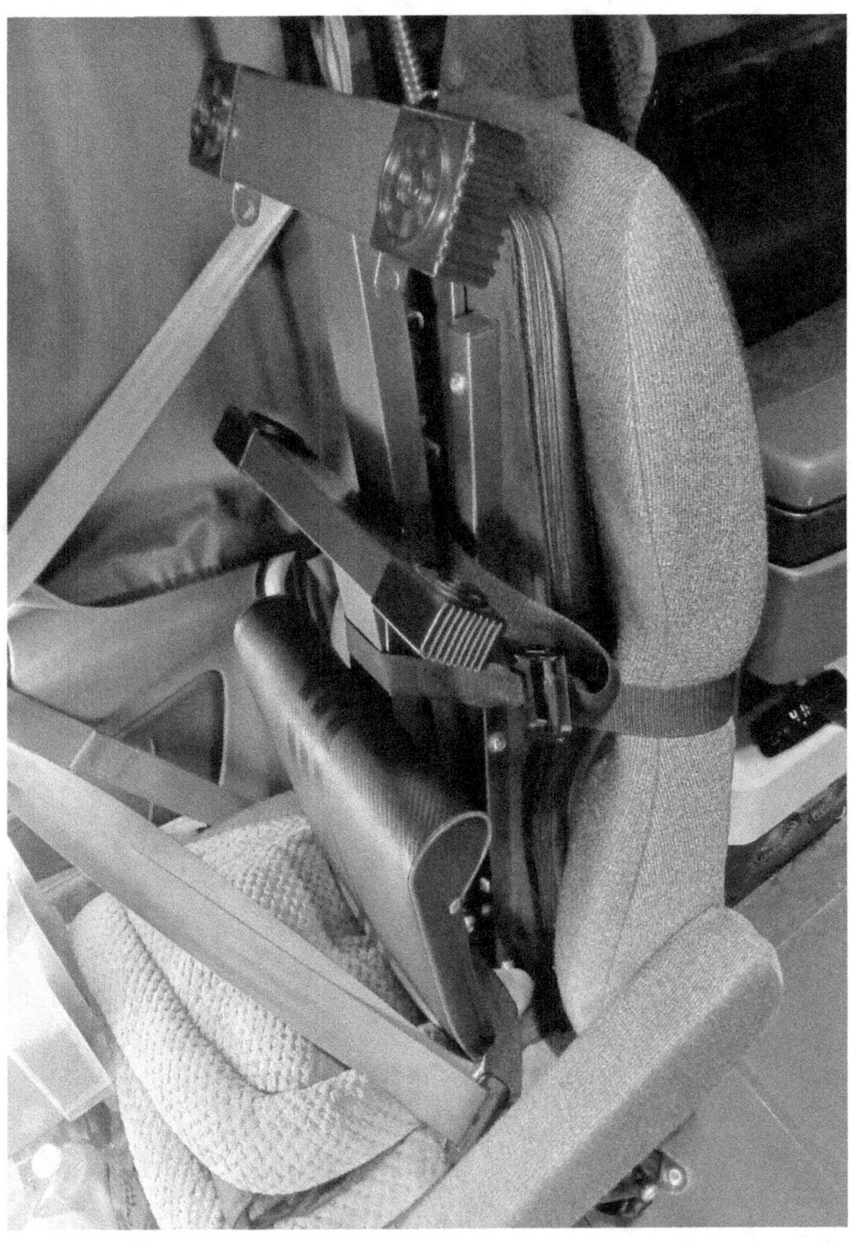

Curling bar set up.

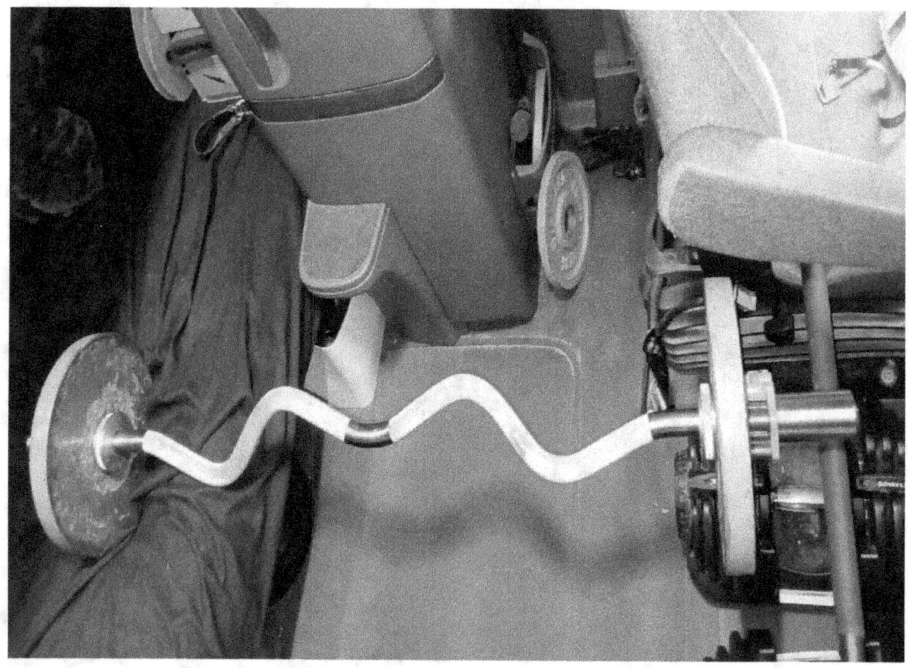

Adjustable dumbbells made by Bowflex.

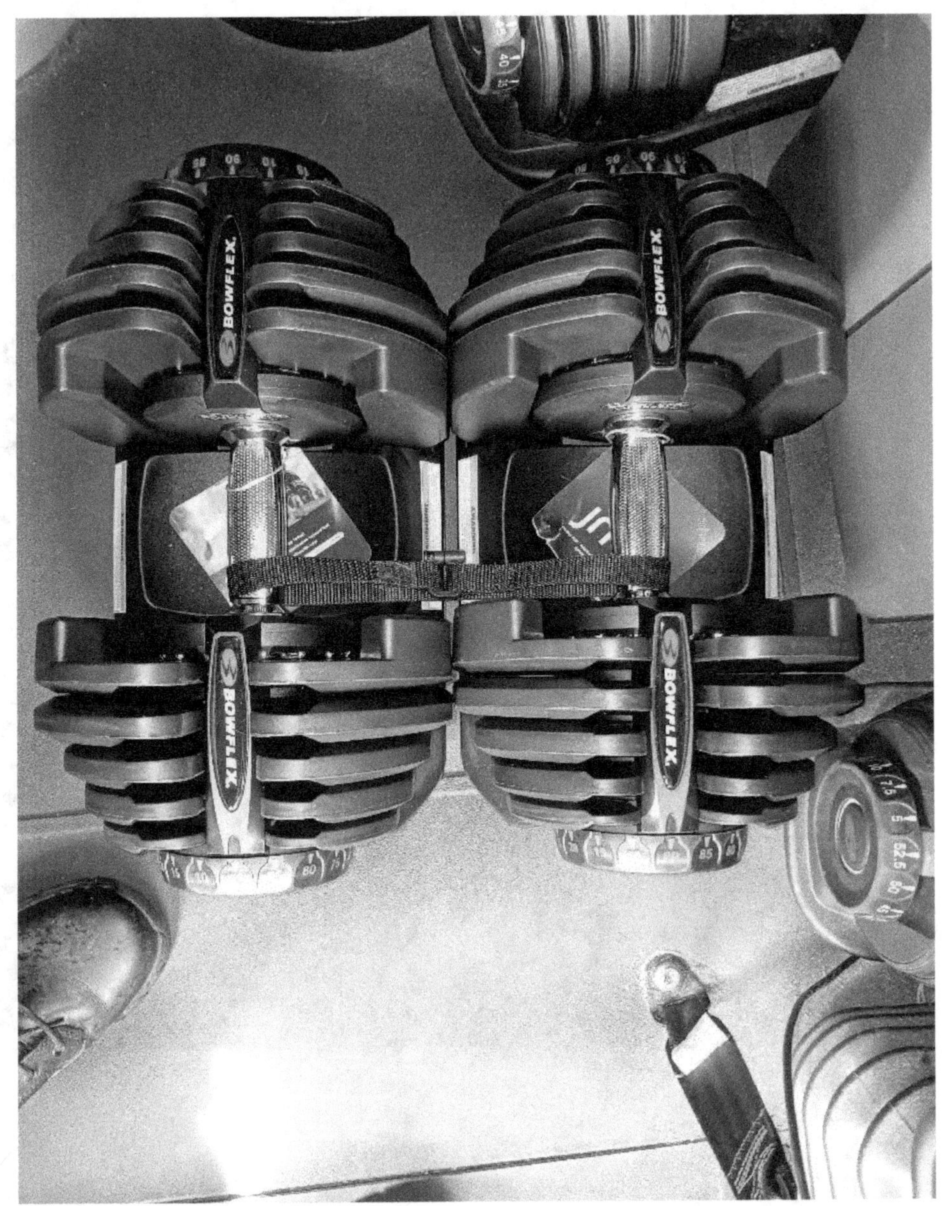

Loading pin with Olympic weights and adjustable dumbbells set up for deadlifts or front squats with the harness.

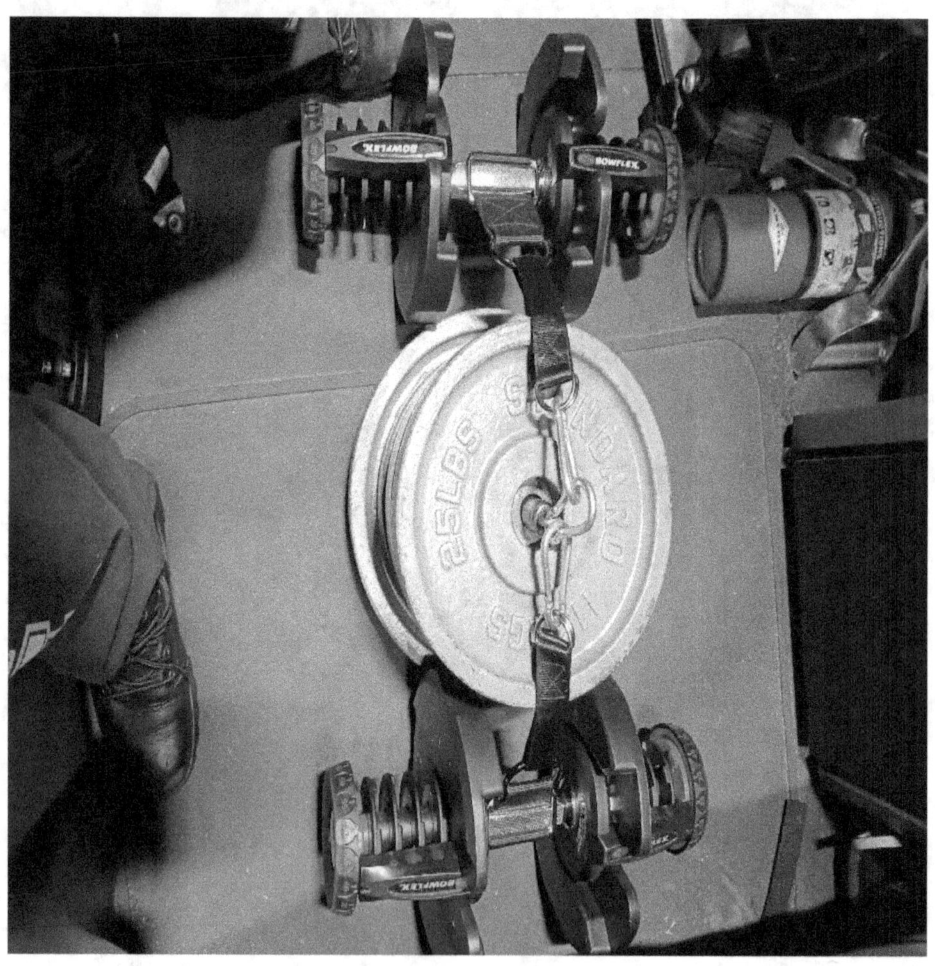

Loading pin and curl bar set up for hammer curls .

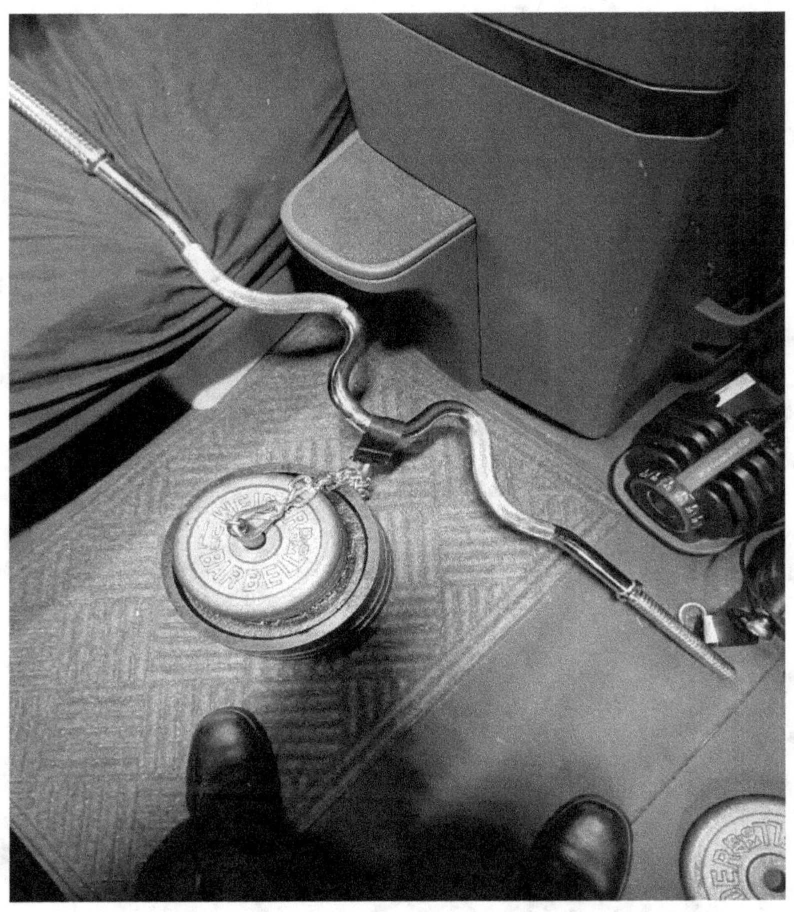

Equipment storage under the bed.

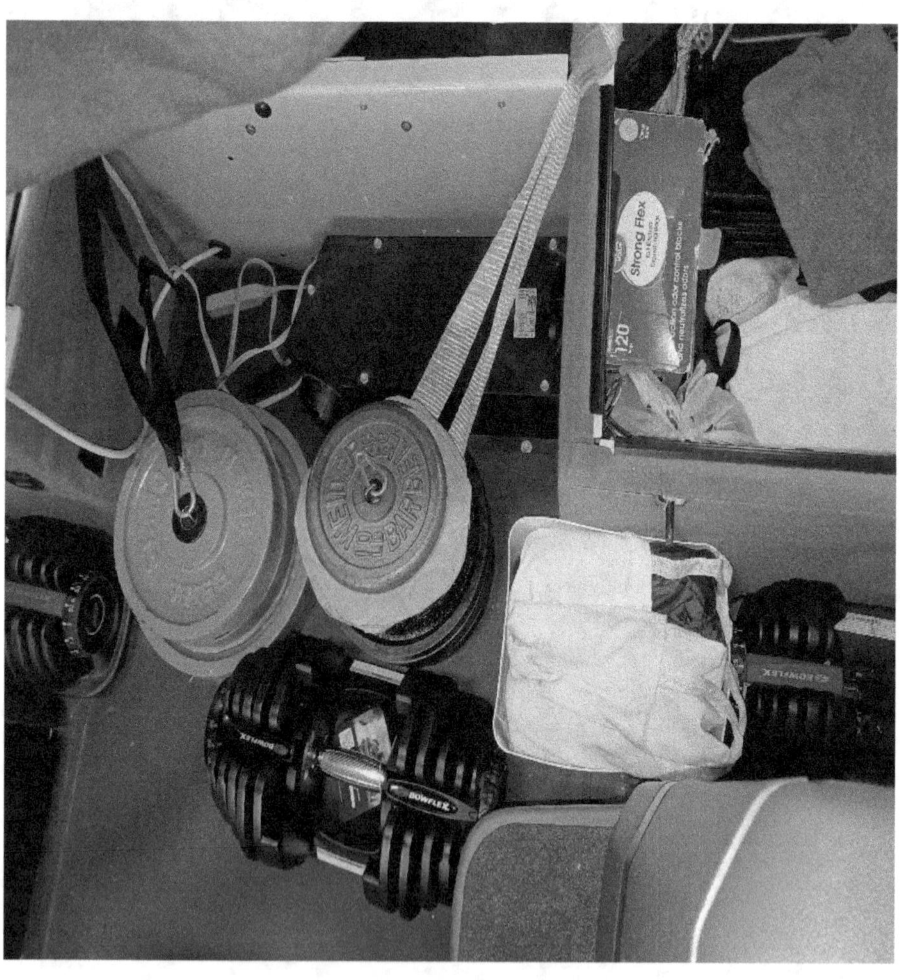

Equipment storage under the bed, with the bed down.

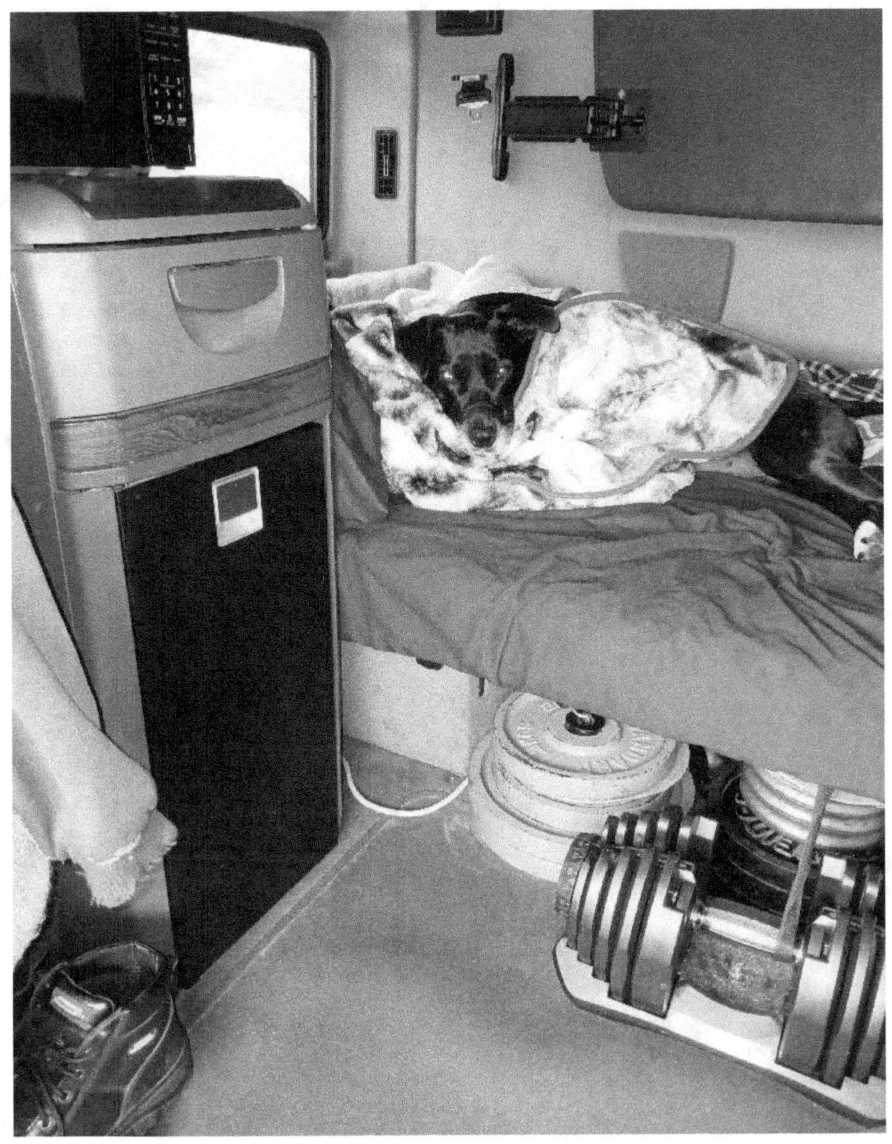

Adjustable chest expander made by Kahegind.

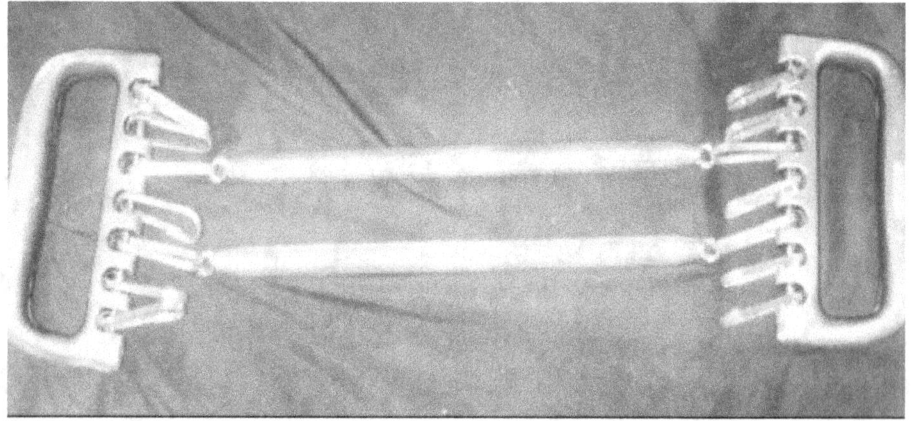

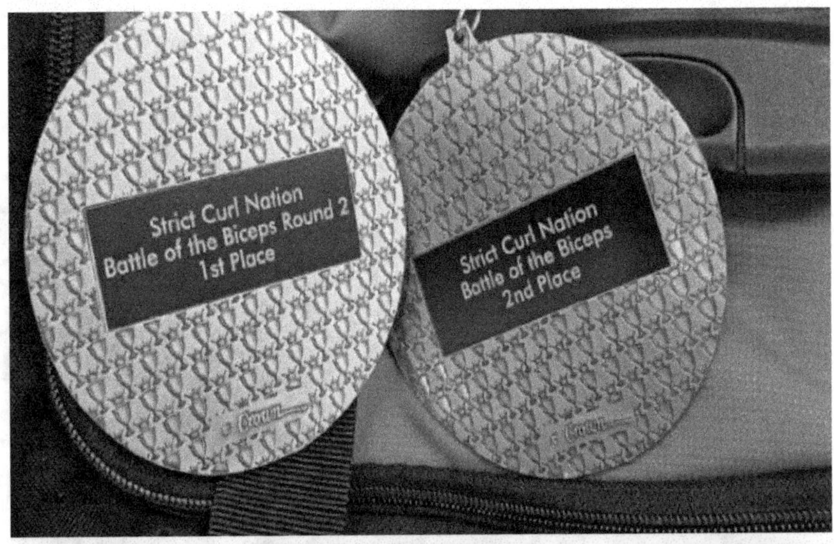

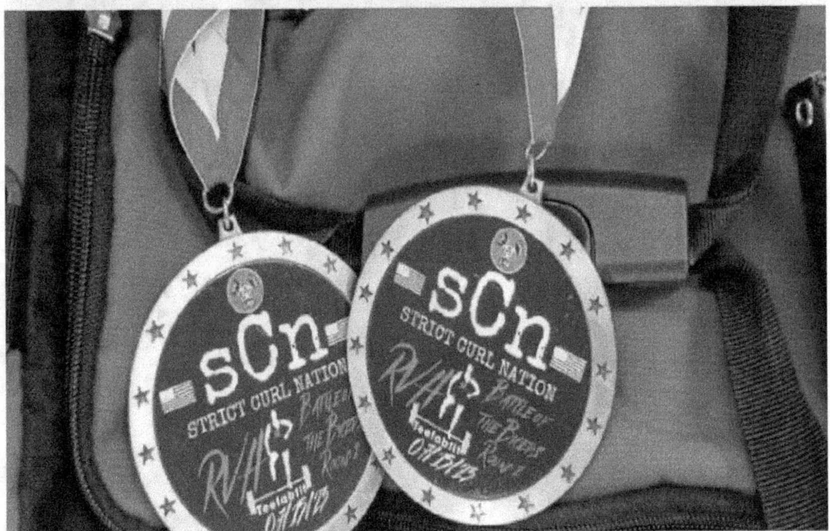

Strict curl competition in 2023

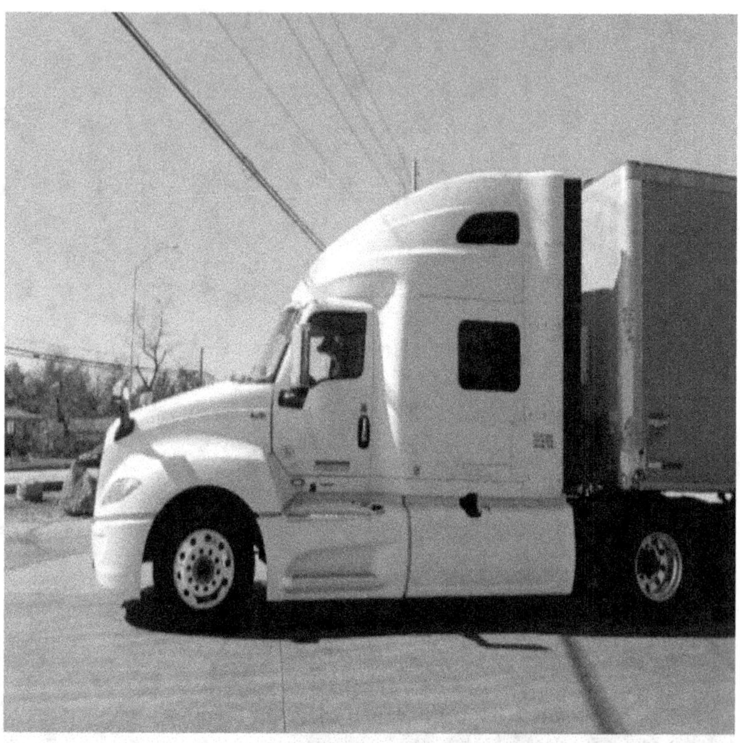

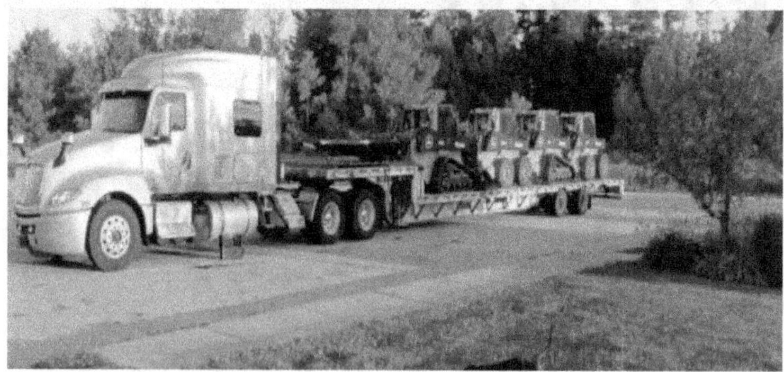

My current truck on top and the bottom picture is a truck I used briefly with a different company.

My little princess ….. Chloe.

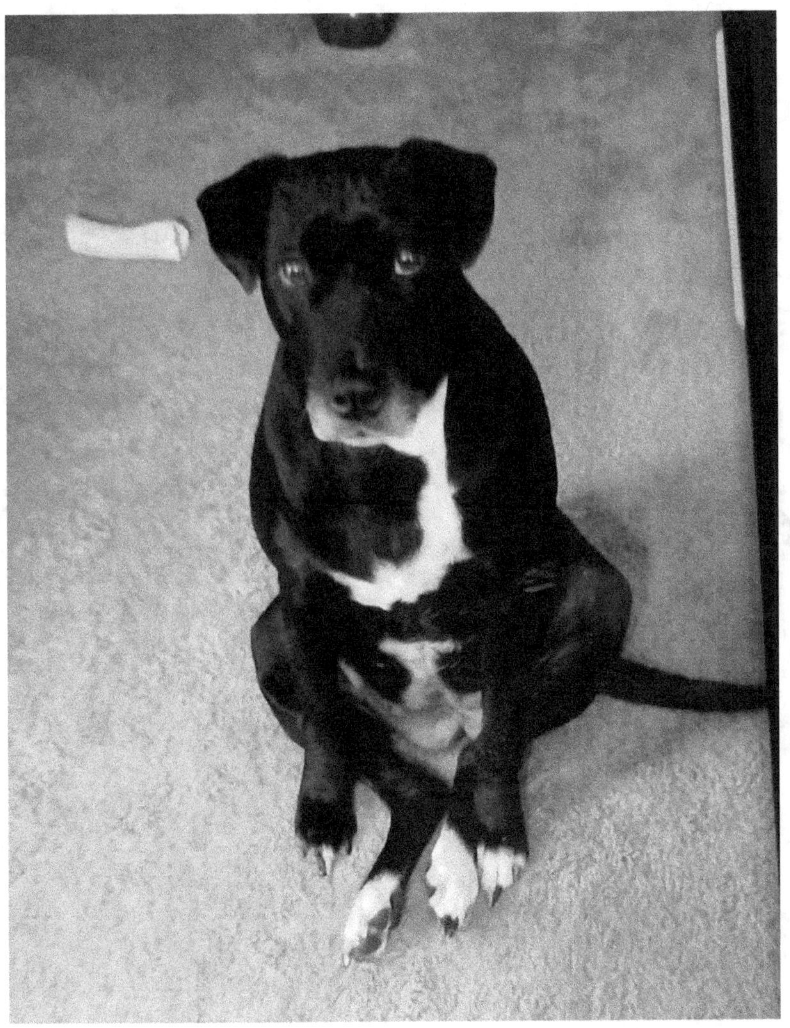

Chloe loves her reset time !!!

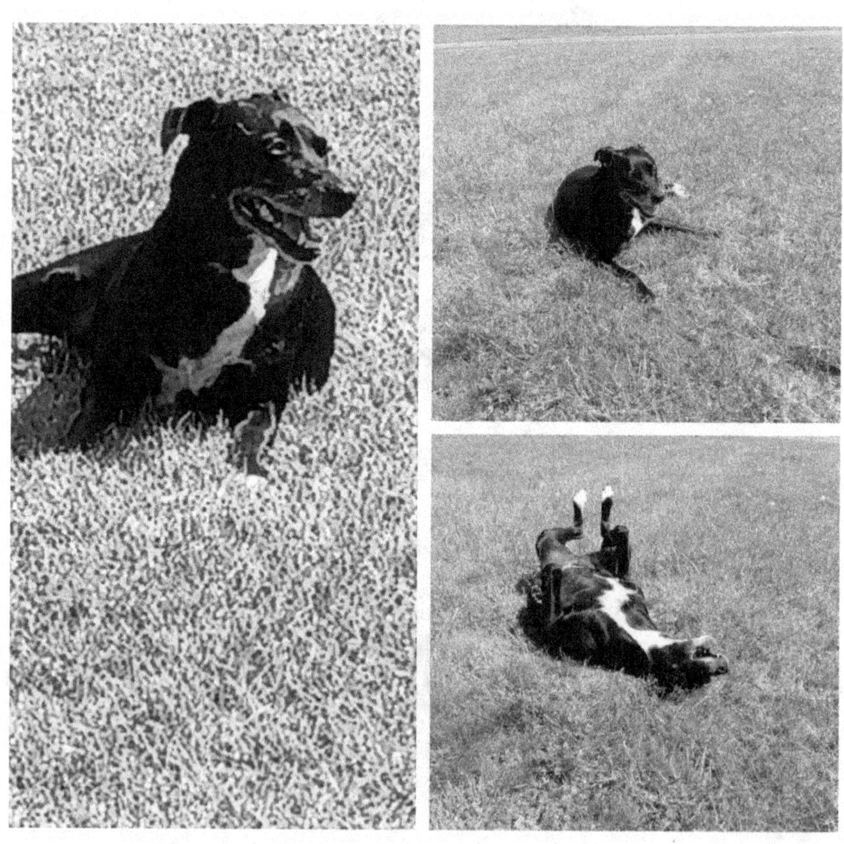

Chloe loves the trucking life, except that one week when it was around zero degrees outside!

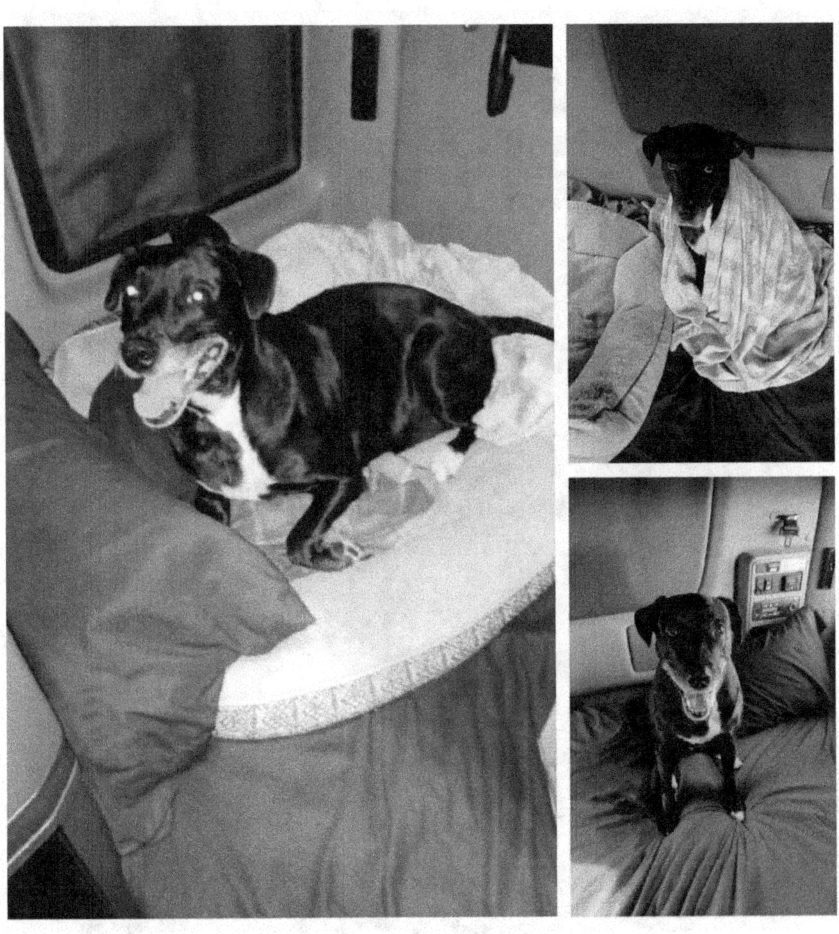

Weekly Carb feasts ;)

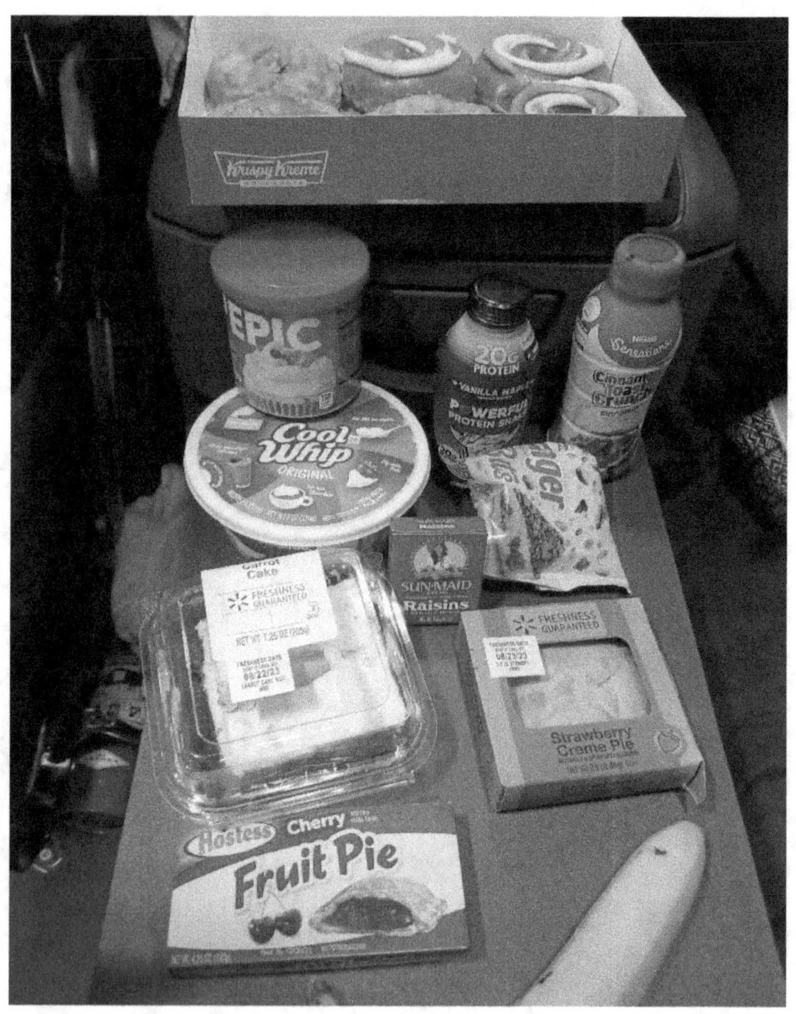

The Adonis Physique

The Adonis physique emphasizes wide shoulders and a small waist, creating a tapered look. The Adonis ratio is 1:1.618, which would make the shoulders 1.618 times bigger than the waist. To have the complete proportionate Adonis physique, other body part measurements come into play.

Waist to Shoulder ratio = 1:1.1618

Wrist to Upper Arm (flexed) ratio = 1:2.5

Calves to Upper Arm (flexed) ratio = 1:1

Wrist to Chest ratio = 1:6.5

Knee to Thigh ratio = 1:1.75

There are certain key muscle groups that would have more of an impact on adding size to the physique and other muscle groups adding more of detail or quality to the physique. The way I would program my training to achieve these measurements are:

Waist to Shoulder ratio = 1:1.1618

-   Decrease bodyfat %.

- Strengthen and tone the abdominals with emphasis on the deepest ab muscle, Transversus Abdominis

- Increase the size of the shoulder muscles with focus on the lateral head

Wrist to Upper Arm (flexed) ratio = 1:2.5

- Increase the size of the Brachialis, Biceps, and Triceps with focus on the long head of the Triceps

Calves to Upper Arm (flexed) ratio = 1:1

- Increase the size of the Brachialis, Biceps, and Triceps with focus on the long head of the Triceps

- Increase the size of both calf muscles, Soleus and Gastrocnemius

Wrist to Chest ratio = 1:6.5

- Increase the size of the Pectoralis major and upper Lat muscles

Knee to Thigh ratio = 1:1.75

- Increase the size of the Quadriceps and Hamstring muscles

There are limited options to perform bodybuilding movements in the truck. These are my go-to movements to increase size to a muscle group.

<u>Quadriceps:</u>

Squats can be performed using dumbbells or using the squat harness with the weight stacks. I can do regular squats or the Bulgarian split squat with either set up. The squat harness imitates performing a front squat with a barbell. The harness set up only allows for squats just above 90 degrees parallel, but puts good emphasis on the quads by keeping more of an upright posture throughout the movement. I can go extremely heavy for 5 reps or do high reps with this set up.

<u>Hamstrings:</u>

Seated leg curls with a TheraBand can be performed but extremely annoying to set up for, so I do not do them at all. I perform Romanian deadlifts with the weight stack and a cambered curl bar cable attachment. I can go extremely heavy for 5 reps or do high reps with this set up.

<u>Calves:</u>

The two calf muscles are trained with heel raises. The Soleus is trained in a seated position and with a bent knee, which I do not do at all. The Gastrocnemius is isolated during standing straight leg heel raises. I use the squat harness with the weight stacks for this movement. I can go extremely heavy, but I rather do higher reps with calves.

<u>Chest:</u>

There is no room for pushups (would have to kick my dog off the bed ….. Princess Chloe does not like that idea!
So, I purchased an adjustable foldable bench, and perform dumbbell presses and/or flys in various positions with emphasis on incline positions.

<u>Back:</u>

The Lat muscles can be trained in many ways on the truck. Pullups off the top bunk, pulldowns using TheraBand, dumbbell pullovers on a slight incline bench, bent over rows with the weight stacks or dumbbells keep the elbows close to the torso. The upper back can be trained with various pull apart movements using the chest expander gadget, bent over rows with dumbbells or the weight stack and a cambered curl bar cable attachment. Keep the elbows flared out to the sides during the rows to isolate more of the upper back.

<u>Traps:</u>

The upper Traps can be isolated by doing standing shrugs.

The middle Traps can be isolated by doing bent over shrugs. Either movement can be performed with dumbbells or the weight stack and a cambered curl bar cable attachment.

<u>Deltoids:</u>

The anterior head can be trained with dumbbell overhead presses, neutral grip incline press or front raises.

The lateral head can be trained with dumbbell upright rows, or lateral raises.

The posterior head can be trained with bent over rows with flared elbows, using either dumbbells or the weight stack and a cambered curl bar cable attachment. I perform pull apart movements using the chest expander gadget instead of bent over dumbbell reverse fly's.

<u>Triceps:</u>

The long head of the Triceps is my focus to add mass to the arm. To emphasize that muscle, I do dumbbell overhead Triceps extension or skull crushers.

The lateral or medial heads can be isolated with various TheraBand Triceps extension.

<u>Biceps:</u>

I use the curling bars, dumbbells and the weight stack and a cambered curl bar cable attachment for biceps training. Changing the grip positions will emphasize different muscles in the arm and forearm. Supinated grip curls, trains the short and long head of the Biceps.

Neutral grip curls, trains the long head of the Biceps, Brachialis and the Brachioradialis. Pronated grip curls, trains the Brachialis and the Brachioradialis.

<u>Forearms:</u>

The forearms can be isolated through wrist curl/extension movements and using grippers. Besides the dumbbells, I have the wrist roller which works better than the dumbbells in my opinion. I also have a set of grippers ranging from 100-350 lbs. in 50 lb. increments. Maybe one day I will use the 300 lb. gripper. The Brachioradialis is a major forearm muscle that also assists in elbow flexion, and it is trained best with neutral or pronated grip curls.

<u>Abs:</u>

Doing regular crunches, reverse crunches and oblique crunches is good enough for me.

Everything I state in this book is my opinion ….. created through my own experiences and my observation from other athletes. There are so many ways to improve strength, muscle, and endurance. You will notice within all sports, that there are a few things that each top athlete all do. Within a golf swing, you have all different takeaways and club head paths, but they all end up with the same body posture upon the moment of impact with a forward shaft lean and downward stroke on the golf ball. That would be a key position to me for consistent ball striking. In billiards, the three keys for consistency are to stay down during the ball strike, stroke the cue straight back/forward and follow through. Simple things to do but most people do not do it, and the skill level remains average at best. Most professional bodybuilders do take steroids and train in a similar fashion, but some have standout body parts compared to the rest of their physique or other bodybuilders. Some examples would be: Tom Platz and his leg development, Arnold Schwarzenegger and his chest development and Dorian Yates and his Lat development. They did different rep ranges but emphasized the stretch position for that body part. They stretched the casing that surrounds the muscle called the fascia, and some would say hyperplasia (muscle splitting) or more room for the muscle to grow. Who knows, but it worked exceptionally well! Tom Platz also did high reps in the stretched position and persevered through the pain of lactic acid build up. In my opinion, he created the best standout body part of all time with the combination of size and definition. Different weight training styles does make a difference in muscle development, as in the difference between Bodybuilders, Powerlifters, and Olympic weightlifters. Bodybuilders have the most pronounced muscle development and have the least strength capability comparable to the other two. Powerlifters have the second most pronounced muscle, but have the most absolute strength. Powerlifters also perform bodybuilding movements along with their strength program to increase their overall body mass. Olympic weightlifters have the least pronounced muscle development of the three but are the most powerful with explosive strength. The last example of muscle development is from track cyclists, who have developed bigger thighs than bodybuilders. They only use concentric contractions, but the high intensity training, creates an extreme muscle pump and the lactic acid accumulation to extremely high levels. This is why I believe in lactic acid accumulation and fascial stretching should be incorporated in weight training to improve the size of a muscle along with heavy weights. Lactic acid is said to increase the production of growth hormone, which is a muscle builder and fat incinerator. My opinion, best bang for your buck to accomplish both fat reduction and build muscle. This is just my take on it, not preaching.

Training Strategies

Timed workouts:

Timed workouts are a great way to formulate a workout program, either for weight loss or muscle building. It will keep you focused, and your effort levels high to push through the uncomfortable feeling of lactic acid accumulation. Anytime you couple workouts that develop lactic acid in the lower and upper body, it truly challenges the cardiovascular system, and will provide a superior fat loss result. This will be the best approach for any fat loss goal. When a muscle group is isolated with a timed workout, it provides the localized growth hormone signal and will improve more of a muscle growth stimulus. My go-to timed workouts are CrossFit workouts from Crossfit.com and the Tabata Protocol (20 seconds work / 10 seconds rest x 8 rounds). They work fantastic for developing a tremendous amount of lactic acid. An example of a CrossFit workout that I do outside the truck is the squat and push-up combo for time. The squats descend in reps from 100 80 60 40 20 and after each set of squats, you do push-ups and they ascend from 10 20 30 40 50.

100 Squats

10 Push-ups

80 Squats

20 Push-ups

60 Squats

30 Push-ups

40 Squats

40 Push-ups

20 Squats

50 Push-ups

I cherry-pick certain CrossFit workouts to do for various reasons. When I first came across their website in 2008, I spent many months just watching the videos. My favorite one at the time was when they had an outside seminar, a female and a male went head-to-head with overhead squats for reps (I forget the weights they used). Well ..... the female won and the males' ego was stuck in the bottom of the hole of his last rep ;) She obviously trained that movement, had impeccable form and was going ATG (ass to grass) on each rep, as he was closer to 90 degrees. One day, I tried a CrossFit workout and afterwards ..... when I caught my breath, I realized a different level of fitness to obtain. Some of the timed workouts I did from Crossfit.com were: Angie, Barbara, Cindy, Diane, and Elizabeth.

Angie: 1 round for time:

100 Pull Ups

100 Push Ups

100 Sit Ups

100 Squats

Barbara: 5 rounds with 3 min rest between rounds for time:

20 Pull Ups

30 Push Ups

40 Sit Ups

50 Squats

Cindy: As many rounds as possible within 20 minutes:

5 Pull Ups

10 Push Ups

15 Squats

Diane: 21/15/9 reps for time:

225 lb. Deadlift

Handstand Push Ups (Substituted with 135 lb. Push Press)

Elizabeth: 21/15/9 reps for time:

135 lb. Squat Cleans

Ring Dips

At the time, I followed the same workout schedule as CrossFit.com, which was a three-day work / one day rest schedule. I did not follow their random workout approach, but would incorporate a strength movement (Deadlift, Overhead Press, Squat) twice throughout the week, with the focus on trying to hit new personal records (PR's) in the 1 rep, 3 rep, or 5 rep range. An example of a week of workouts would be:

Monday: Cindy

Tuesday: Deadlift training with focus on 3 reps

Wednesday: Diane

Thursday: Rest

Friday: Barbara

Saturday: Overhead Press training with focus on 5 reps

Sunday: Elizabeth

Monday: Rest

I do not remember how I stumbled across their website, but extremely grateful I did. I must have watched all the videos and read their articles they posted during that time. I achieved an overall strength and fitness level that bodybuilding routines could not come close too.

Isometric Training:

On the truck, I only use isometric training to improve my strict curl strength. Resistance on a muscle, that is closer to a 1 rep max of force, will emphasize neural recruitment to that muscle or movement. It will strengthen all structures involved in the movement. The Bones/Ligaments/Tendons will become denser, the Nervous system will improve its density/connections, and speed/bursts of signals to the muscle. I use various timed contractions: 5 sec, 10 sec, 30 sec, 60 sec. Each one will improve the other times in some way. If I hit a plateau of my 5 second times with a certain weight, I would focus on improving my 10, 30 or 60 second times with a certain weight. That usually will help blast through any plateau. The nervous system gets fatigued too, so there are times that I would just take 5 days off from any heavy resistance to let my nervous system recover. With me, neural fatigue drains my whole body/mind, but muscle fatigue recovers extremely fast.

Strength and Bodybuilding:

For strength, if you systematically increase weight within the 3 or 5 rep ranges, the strength levels will gradually improve for that muscle or movement over time. For bodybuilding, more time under tension is needed to increase metabolic stress (lactic acid development) and overall muscle fiber fatigue. The CrossFit workouts changed my perception of what training should be. When I started incorporating timed workouts and the CrossFit rep schemes with bodybuilding movements, I seen more overall muscle development. You can use any set interval time for work/rest as in the Tabata Protocol, or a certain number of reps to get done as fast as possible and rest when needed. Super strict form is not going to be established throughout the entire number of reps but it should be as close as possible. Here are a couple of variations for isolation or compound bodybuilding movements:

The 5-rep max / 35-rep drop set:

Incorporate a 5-rep max to the movement before the high rep sets. It primes the nervous system to the muscles, which would improve the strength levels for that movement. This is how the workout would look like:

- Set 1 – warm up sets, than sets that work up to a 5rep max

- Rest 3-5 minutes

- Set 2 – subtract 10-20 lbs. from the 5-rep max and do 35 reps. Most likely, you will be unable to complete the 35 reps but do as many as possible, rest for 3 deep breaths than do as many reps as you can again. If still unable to complete the 35 reps, rest for 3 deep breaths and do as many reps as you can. Continue until you reach 35 reps.

- Rest 1 minute

- Set 3 – subtract 10-20 lbs. from the previous round of 35 reps. Now complete 35 reps with the decreased weight. If unable to complete the 35 reps, rest for 3 deep breaths and do as many reps as you can. If still unable to complete the 35 reps, rest for 3 deep breaths and do as many reps as you can. Continue until you reach 35 reps.

- Rest 1 minute

- Set 4 - subtract 10-20 lbs. from the previous round of 35 reps. Continue the previous process until you can do 35 reps without resting.

The 5-rep max / 35-rep scheme I just explained, covers all muscle fiber types, the nervous system, and the cardiovascular system. *One of my favorite ways of training!*

The Tabata Protocol:

The Tabata protocol is 8 rounds of 20 seconds of all out work and 10 seconds of rest. It is a great method to incorporate on the truck due to time constraints. You can also incorporate a 5-rep max to the movement prior of the Tabata or do it on its own. I am currently using a modified Tabata protocol with 5 rounds of 20 seconds of all out work and 10 seconds of rest. I keep the same weight with each movement or muscle until I can achieve more than 35 reps within the 5 rounds. This approach improves size and strength. I also use a weight with a 50 rep goal, which improves size and endurance.

I have trained within various rep schemes throughout the years and this is how I see each one has improved my body:

Isometrics:

- Improved quality of muscle contraction

- Stability of the movement

- Muscle tone

- Increased strength near joint angle of movement

Low Reps of 1-5:

- Increased absolute strength

- Minimal muscle definition

- Overall muscle thickness

Moderate Reps of 6-15:

- Increased strength

- Good muscle growth and definition

High Reps of 15-50:

- Good muscle definition

- Increased vascularity

I trained in those rep schemes from teenage years to my 30's, with more focus on 10 reps and lower. I just did the normal protein drink and carbs post workout, and ate the normal 3 times a day. When I was mid 30's or so, I wanted to get as big and strong as possible. Did not care about body composition, so I followed the 5x5 program and ate to grow. My consistent lunch was the Burger King's A1 thick burger with large fries and soda. I became ridiculously strong but the waist size grew along with it. I was up to a 36-inch pants that were getting snug. I am not a big framed character so that was damn fat. Went to tie my shoes one day for work and had to exhale to do it, cause that fat ass belly got in the way. Loved my strength levels but had to say goodbye to those A1 thick burgers. I switched training styles for a couple of years than went back to the 5x5 program to increase strength. Then finally for the first time, I injured myself.

Last rep of the last set of the last exercise ….. I felt something give in my lower back and an electric shock shot up my spine. Felt like a vertebral disc blew out the back of my spine. It was during T-Bar rows ….. I dropped the weight, fell to my knees, hung out there for a while with the "WTF!!!" thought going through my mind, then crawled into the house (gym was in the garage). Every muscle tightened up near my lower spine within the next few minutes. No reason to describe the pain levels that accompanied that issue. Chiropractor visits with spinal adjustments were needed to take the pressure off the compressed nerves. It took about two to three weeks' time for my body to relax and reduce that protective reaction of tense muscles around the injured area. Those next few weeks were horrible, since I had to continue to work every day. I had responsibilities that had to be maintained. I owned/operated a landscaping business (one man crew), owned/operated a vending machine business (one man crew), and Physical Therapist Assistant on the weekends. That injury had no negative effect when in a standing position except just a constant tightness around the lower back region. It only interfered if I had to bend down or squat down. My lower back wanted to stay in its fixed position. Surprising enough, landscaping and the vending machine businesses were not that much of an issue. I had stand on lawnmowers, so when I had to pick something up or when opening/closing the trailer door was the main issue. Doing the therapy job was horrible ….. with the constant up/down you must do to remove wheelchair leg rests or put on/off ankle weights, etc….. Well, after the back issue went away, I realized I cannot let that happen again. Refrained from heavy weights and decided to try something I never thought about. Get as shredded as possible like Bruce Lee. Changed my diet to proteins / fats, and high rep movements of 50-250 reps. Performed a lot of CrossFit.com timed workouts multiple times a day while experimenting with various combinations of protein / fat meals (not really counting calories at this time). I dropped 40 pounds in 9 weeks. My guess would be a good amount of water weight, fat, and I am sure muscle too. To whom that has never did a CrossFit.com timed workout before ….. post workout ….. I am laying on the ground for about 5-10 minutes, and the sweat is coating your body. You go from a feeling of complete exhaustion to 20-25 minutes later feeling great. I continued to adjust my diet and came across a protein and fat combination that incorporated peanut butter and cool whip. I love peanut butter! The only downside was it carried extra calories. So, I decided, if I was going to eat it, I had to earn it. The workout I chose on a consistent basis was, partial rep pull-ups and partial rep flat bench with 95 lbs. Wanted to eliminate the smaller muscle groups and keep constant tension on the pecs and lats. Started with 50 total reps each, performed with the rest / pause method. The pull-ups were the grind movement and the bench was the active recovery. I would eat that peanut butter and protein meal afterwards. Within a few days, I decided to do 5 rounds of the 50 reps each. You got to earn that meal. Did that for a week or two, but all I wanted to do was eat more of that protein and peanut butter meal. It was ridiculously delicious!!! ….. 5 rounds of 50 reps each (rest/pause) x 4 times a day was born. The amount of calories for the day was 3500-4000. My daily schedule was:

- Wake up and do 20 minutes on the stationary bike.

- 5 rounds x 50 reps each of pull-ups and presses

- Eat protein and peanut butter meal

- Go do the landscaping business x 3 to 4 lawns. The lawns were small and landscaping accounts were within the community complex.

- 5 rounds x 50 reps each of pull-ups and presses

- Eat protein and peanut butter meal

- 3 to 4 lawns

- 5 rounds x 50 reps each of pull-ups and presses

- Eat protein and peanut butter meal

- 3 to 4 lawns
- 5 rounds x 50 reps each of pull-ups and presses

- Eat protein and peanut butter meal

As you can tell, the days started early and ended late. I am a very regimented character, but also goal oriented. Even though it was a high calorie diet, I lost more weight and became more muscular than ever before. I would have continued doing that workout / diet combo but learned the hard way about peanut butter. Peanuts are high in Lectins and can cause gut issues. The abdominal pain it caused one day, had me on the floor in the fetal position. Say goodbye to peanut butter. I tried almond butter and other types of nut butters, but nothing compared to that peanut butter. So sad! Don't recall how many weeks of that schedule was performed, but I was not "overtrained" like the experts said would happen. Experts also said a no carb diet is bad for endurance. At that time, I could have outworked anyone ….. well at least I felt that way. I had endless amounts of energy before/during/after workouts and throughout the day. Never had energy crashes, and I still do a protein / fat diet till this day. The next experiment was to increase arm and shoulder size. A buddy of mine had big biceps and he did bicep curls every day. I took it up a notch and did it multiple times a day. I put a pair of 30 lb. dumbbells in my bedroom and started with a couple rounds a day of bilateral hammer curls x 50 reps, single dumbbell bilateral overhead triceps extension x 100 reps, and blue TheraBand shoulder movement (Pull apart, bottom position shoulder lateral raise, PNF D2 flexion). They all were done in the rest / pause method. At first, the number of reps took multiple rest pause sessions to complete. Weeks later, I was able to complete over 50 reps of bilateral hammer curls without putting down the dumbbells (rested with them in my hands), and moved the reps to 75. I was able to do 70+ reps before resting on the overhead triceps extension and 100+ reps on the bottom position shoulder lateral raises which I bumped to 250 reps when I performed them on their own. I also increased the number of times I would do those 3 exercises throughout the day to 10+ times a day. Every time I walked in my bedroom, I would bust out a round. I became obsessed, but the arm and shoulder development matched my effort level. The Brachioradialis of the forearm, long head of the Biceps, Brachialis, longhead of the Triceps and all three heads of the Deltoids became extremely developed. What that workout did not improve was the short head of the bicep which is demonstrated in a front double bicep pose. Do not have to tell you which way I always flexed the bicep. Later in life I did a similar approach using a supinated grip curl and fixed that issue. I have achieved overall muscular development and vascularity through high rep / high frequency training than any other type of methods. Do not confuse muscular development with massive muscle size. My description of muscular development is Moderate amounts of size with extreme definition and shape. Quality over quantity!!! Still bigger than most at any gym. Every training and diet method / ideology taught me different things on how my body responded. Present day within the truck, I do brief workouts using various versions of the Tabata Protocol, the 5 rep/35 rep workout, or a timed workout. The only strength specific training I do is to improve my strict curl. I keep my diet on the lower end to make sure I do not accumulate any fat. I'm trying not to gain weight so I can compete in the strict curl competition without having to go up in a weight class. I am striving to break that world record. Since my diet is low in calories, it forces the body to utilize fat for energy and the glycogen stores within the muscle. Once every 5 to 7 days, I have a carbohydrate feast of 3500 - 4500 calories. Anything goes, packages of cookies, pancakes, pies, shakes and ice cream. It is a beautiful thing and beneficial. It ramps up the metabolism, restores glycogen within the muscles, and puts a big smile on the face with no regrets!

Throughout my younger years, lifting weights progressively became a strong passion, and has remained so till this day. I Love It! Every few months, I like to emphasize different aspects of training. Hypothetically, if I wanted to achieve the Adonis physique, and do so while trucking, this is how I would change my training and diet accordingly.

The Adonis physique, body part ratios:

Waist to Shoulder ratio = 1:1.1618

Wrist to Upper Arm (flexed) ratio = 1:2.5

Calves to Upper Arm (flexed) ratio = 1:1

Wrist to Chest ratio = 1:6.5

Knee to Thigh ratio = 1:1.75

First, I take my measurements and compare them to the list above. That would give me an objective list of muscles that need to increase in size and if I also need to lose weight. If my measurements show me that I do need to have a smaller waist and/or bigger muscles, I would adjust my training and diet accordingly. I would leave my diet the same at the beginning and see if my weight reduces by just adding in upper/lower body timed workouts. I would also add in training to increase any specific body part, how I explained earlier in this book. Here is an outline of my weekly schedule for work and training:

Monday

- Weight loss workout before I start my day

- Drive to destination / deliver / drive back to distribution center

- More stops today so I just do the one weight loss workout.

Tuesday

- Weight loss workout before I start my day

- Drive to destination / deliver / drive back to distribution center

- There is down time during my work hours to go off duty and perform a Tabata for muscle gain. Tabata's are only 4 minutes in duration. Use the Tabata for any of the smaller muscles of the arm, shoulder, or calves.

Wednesday

- More stops today so I make it a rest day.

Thursday

- 5-rep max / 35-rep scheme for the chest, back or thigh muscles before I start my day

- Drive to destination / deliver / drive back to distribution center

- There is down time during my work hours to go off duty and perform a Tabata for muscle gain. Tabata's are only 4 minutes in duration. Use the Tabata for

any of the smaller muscles of the arm, shoulder, or calves.

Friday

- Weight loss workout before I start my day

- Drive to destination / deliver / drive back to distribution center

- There is down time during my work hours to go off duty and perform a Tabata for muscle gain. Tabata's are only 4 minutes in duration. Use the Tabata for any of the smaller muscles of the arm, shoulder, or calves.

Saturday (34 hour reset)

- 5-rep max / 35-rep scheme for the chest, back or thigh muscles

- Tabata Protocol using an isolation movement

- During the 34 hour reset, I could add a weight loss workout, or perform multiple muscle building workouts. Depends on other responsibilities.

Sunday (34 hour reset)

- 5-rep max / 35-rep scheme for the chest, back or thigh muscles

- Tabata Protocol using an isolation movement

- During the 34 hour reset, I could add a weight loss workout, or perform multiple muscle building workouts. Depends on other responsibilities.

I am not being specific on the body parts worked for the muscle building, as they will always change as the measurements improve and the need to focus more on other muscles. The Tabata protocol does not seem to cause any issues with being able to train the same muscle multiple times a week. The 5-rep max / 35-rep scheme is more intense and I would take at least a day or two before doing another specific muscle building workout to that muscle. On the other hand, I might or might not work that same muscle in a weight loss workout the following day. I assess on pre-workout basis. I could also do a full body workout 2 to 3 days a week and walk a certain distance other days. There are always multiple options to choose from.

Even though the space is limited in the truck, I can accomplish almost a complete bodybuilding program.

Bodyweight Movements:

- Squats or Bulgarian Split Squat

- Heel Raises

- Pull-ups

- Push-ups

- Sit-ups

Dumbbell Movements:

- Thruster: is a great overall full body compound movement that will build strength, muscle, and burn fat.

- Front Squat or Bulgarian Split Squat

- Romanian Deadlift

- Heel Raises

- Pull-ups

- Bent Over Rows

- Bench Press is limited to using the bed as the surface, but I highly recommend the Incline Foldable Bench

- Strict Press, Push Press, or Push Jerk

- Front, Side, and Rear Delt Raises

- Bicep Curls

- Triceps Extensions

- Forearm Curls/Extensions

There are many variations with sets and reps within a workout. Adjust the sets and reps for each body part, movement, or fitness goals. Progressive resistance is a major factor to improve strength and size, and most likely, you will have limited resistance on the truck. Once that happens, reduce the rest periods between sets, and/or add more sets. Common rep schemes are:

5 sets of 5 repetitions, I would recommend for strength and size:

- Use on compound movements to improve overall strength and size with the least amount of time needed. Start with 3-to-5-minute rest periods and reduce the rest periods by 30 seconds once you reached the max resistance you have on the truck. Use the same weight for all 5 sets and on the 5th set, do as many reps as possible. If you can get 7 or so reps, add 5-10 pounds. If you can get 10 or more reps, add 10-20 pounds. There will be a trial-and error period. Do not add weight until you can at least get all 5 sets with 5 repetitions.

4 sets of 8 to 12 repetitions, I would recommend for more emphasis on size:

- Use on compound or isolation movements. Start with 2 minute rest periods and reduce the rest periods by 30 seconds once you reached the max resistance you have on the truck. You can also use the 5-rep max / 35-rep scheme or the Tabata protocol using an isolation movement, instead of the 4 sets of 8-12 reps.

Workouts I would recommend for weight loss:

- The CrossFit workout named "Fran" using dumbbells: 21/15/9 reps of dumbbell thrusters / pullups for time:

- The CrossFit workout: squat/push-up combo for time: 100/10, 80/20, 60/30, 40/40, 20/50

Go on Crossfit.com, look in the exercise section, and pick out workouts to your liking.

- Tabata Protocol using any compound movement

I have given options to get anyone started and make progress for years while on the road. Good luck on your journey ….. set the goal, then go get it!

Notes